MW01489951

INTRODUCTION

ACXION Pills, additionally known as Phentermine, are a form of prescription medication that acts as an urge for food suppressant. They belong to a class of drugs called sympathomimetic amines, which are similar to amphetamines. ACXION Pills work by stimulating the discharge of chemical substances within the brain that manipulate hunger and satiety, in the long run decreasing appetite and promoting weight loss. But how precisely do those pills attain such tremendous consequences? Let's take a closer take a look at the mechanisms in the back of their effectiveness. When you devour ACXION Pills, the active component, Phentermine hydrochloride, acts as a stimulant at the critical apprehensive system. This stimulation results in the suppression of appetite, making you feel much less hungry during the day. By curtailing your cravings and reducing the choice to eat, ACXION Pills assist you stay on course together with your weight reduction dreams.

HOW TO APPLY PHENTERMINE HCL

Take this medicine by mouth as directed through your medical doctor, usually once an afternoon, 1 hour earlier than breakfast or 1 to 2 hours after breakfast. If wished, your doctor may alter your dose to take a small dose up to a few times an afternoon. Carefully follow your health practitioner's instructions. Taking this medicine overdue inside the day may motive hassle drowsing (insomnia). If you're the use of sustained-release tablets, the dose is commonly taken once an afternoon before breakfast or at least 10 to fourteen hours earlier than bedtime. Swallow the medicine entire. Do now not crush or bite sustained-launch pills. Doing so can release the entire drug right away, increasing the hazard of side outcomes. If you are the use of the capsules made to dissolve inside the mouth, the dose is commonly taken as soon as a day within the morning, without or with food. First, dry your hands earlier than managing the tablet. Place your dose on pinnacle of the tongue till it dissolves, then swallow it without or with water.

The dosage and period of remedy are based totally on your clinical condition and reaction to treatment. Your medical doctor will alter the dose to locate the great dose for you. Discuss the dangers and blessings, and the length of phentermine remedy, along with your physician. To get the maximum gain, take this remedy regularly, precisely as prescribed, and for so long as directed through your medical doctor. To help you recollect, take it at the same time(s) each day.

If you unexpectedly stop using this medicinal drug, you could have withdrawal signs (consisting of melancholy, extreme tiredness). To assist prevent withdrawal; your doctor can also decrease your dose slowly. Withdrawal is much more likely if you have used phentermine for a long time or in excessive doses. Tell your doctor or pharmacist proper away if you have withdrawal.

Though it enables many humans, this medication may additionally occasionally purpose addiction. This threat can be better if you have a substance use disease (which includes overuse of or dependancy to drugs/alcohol). Do now not increase your dose, take it extra often, or use it for an extended time than prescribed.

Properly stop the drugs while so directed.

This medicine may forestall running well after you have been taking it for some weeks. Talk with your physician if this medication stops running well. Do no longer growth the dose unless directed through your doctor. Your physician may also direct you to stop taking this medicine.

SIDE EFFECTS

Dizziness, dry mouth, trouble drowsing, irritability, nausea, vomiting, diarrhea, or constipation can also occur. If any of these results closing or get worse, inform your health practitioner or pharmacist right away.

Remember that this medication has been prescribed because your physician has judged that the advantage to you is extra than the risk of aspect effects. Many people using this medication do no longer have severe side effects.

This remedy might also improve your blood stress. Check your blood stress regularly and tell your medical doctor if the results are high.

Tell your doctor proper away if you have any severe aspect consequences, which includes: rapid/abnormal/pounding heartbeat, intellectual/temper modifications (consisting of agitation, uncontrolled anger, hallucinations, and nervousness), uncontrolled muscle movements, change in sexual ability/interest.

Stop taking this medication and get scientific help proper away when you have any very serious side results, along with: severe headache, trouble speaking, seizure, weakness on one side of the body, vision modifications (consisting of blurred imaginative and prescient).

This drug may additionally rarely cause serious (once in a while fatal) lung or coronary heart issues (pulmonary hypertension, coronary heart valve troubles). The danger may additionally growth with longer use of this medication and use of this drug along side other appetite-suppressant tablets/natural products. Stop taking this medication and get medical help proper away if you have any very extreme facet consequences, consisting of: chest pain, trouble respiration with exercising, reduced ability to workout, fainting, swelling of the legs/ankles/feet. A very critical allergic reaction to this drug is uncommon. However, get scientific assist right away in case you observe any symptoms of a severe hypersensitivity, which include: rash, itching/swelling (especially of the face/tongue/throat), extreme dizziness, problem respiration.

This isn't always a complete listing of feasible aspect results. If you notice different results now not listed above, touch your doctor or pharmacist.

PRECAUTIONS

Before taking this remedy, inform your health practitioner or pharmacist if you are allergic to it; or to some other sympathomimetic amines (together with decongestants inclusive of pseudoephedrine, stimulants including amphetamine, appetite suppressants such as diethylpropion); or when you have any other hypersensitive reactions. This product may also include inactive substances that could cause allergic reactions or other troubles. Talk for your pharmacist for more information.

Before the usage of this remedy, tell your doctor or pharmacist your medical records, especially of: diabetes, excessive blood strain, glaucoma, non-public or circle of relatives records of a substance use disorder (which includes overuse of or dependancy to pills/alcohol), heart sickness (along with chest pain, heart attack, heart murmur, fast/irregular heartbeat, coronary heart valve problems), mental/temper problems (which includes depression, thoughts of suicide, excessive anxiety/agitation), high blood stress inside the lungs (pulmonary high blood pressure), stroke, overactive thyroid (hyperthyroidism), kidney disorder, seizures.

This drug can also make you dizzy or blur your vision. It might also rarely make you drowsy. Alcohol or marijuana (hashish) can make you more dizzy or drowsy. Do no longer force, use equipment, or do anything that wishes alertness or clear imaginative and prescient until you may do it thoroughly. Avoid alcoholic liquids. Talk for your medical doctor if you are the use of marijuana (cannabis).

If you've got diabetes, check your blood sugar often as directed and percentage the effects along with your physician. Your physician may additionally want to alter your diabetes remedy for the duration of treatment with this drug. If you are using the drugs made to dissolve within the mouth, your medicinal drug may additionally comprise aspartame. If you have phenylketonuria (PKU) or some other situation that requires you to limit/avoid aspartame (or phenylalanine) to your weight loss program, ask your physician or pharmacist about the use of this remedy properly.

Before having surgical operation, tell your health practitioner or dentist about all the products you use (along with pharmaceuticals, nonprescription pills, and natural products).

Older adults may be at greater chance for dizziness and high blood pressure whilst using this drug.

This medicinal drug needs to now not be used all through pregnancy. It may harm an unborn child. If you're pregnant or think you will be pregnant, inform your physician right away.

This drug may also bypass into breast milk and could have undesirable results on a nursing toddler. Breastfeeding isn't advocated at the same time as the usage of this drug. Consult your medical doctor before breastfeeding.

INTERACTIONS

Drug interactions may alternate how your medicinal drugs paintings or growth your risk for severe side consequences. This record does now not comprise all viable drug interactions. Keep a listing of all the products you use (which includes prescription/nonprescription pills and herbal merchandise) and share it with your physician and pharmacist. Do not start, prevent, or trade the dosage of any medicines without your physician's approval.

This drug must now not be used with certain medicinal drugs due to the fact very extreme interactions may occur. If you're taking or have taken different urge for food-suppressant pills within the beyond 12 months (which include diethylpropion, ephedra/ma huang), tell your physician or pharmacist before starting this medication.

Taking MAO inhibitors with this remedy might also motive a critical (possibly fatal) drug interaction. Avoid taking MAO inhibitors (isocarboxazid, linezolid, metaxalone, methylene blue, moclobemide, phenelzine, procarbazine, rasagiline, safinamide, selegiline, tranylcypromine) throughout remedy with this medication. Most MAO inhibitors need to also not be taken for 2 weeks earlier than treatment with this medicinal drug. Ask your health practitioner while to begin or prevent taking this medication.

Some products that can have interaction with this drug are: excessive blood stress medication (which include guanethidine, methyldopa), phenothiazines (along with prochlorperazine, chlorpromazine), other stimulants (which includes amphetamines, methylphenidate, street pills consisting of cocaine or MDMA/"ecstasy").

Tell your medical doctor or pharmacist if you are taking other products that motive drowsiness including opioid pain or cough relievers (including codeine, hydrocodone), alcohol, marijuana (cannabis), drugs for sleep or tension (which include alprazolam, lorazepam, zolpidem), muscle relaxants (such as carisoprodol, cyclobenzaprine), or antihistamines (which include cetirizine, diphenhydramine).

Check the labels on all of your drug treatments (including allergic reaction or cough-and-bloodless merchandise) due to the fact they may include elements that purpose drowsiness. Ask your pharmacist approximately the use of those merchandise competently. Some products have ingredients that could enhance your heart rate or blood pressure. Tell your pharmacist what products you're using, and ask the way to use them competently (mainly cough-and-cold products or weight-reduction plan aids).

Caffeine can boom the facet outcomes of this medicinal drug. Avoid drinking massive amounts of liquids containing caffeine (coffee, tea, colas) or consuming massive amounts of chocolate.

This medication can also intrude with certain medical/lab assessments (which includes mind scan for Parkinson's sickness), in all likelihood causing fake check consequences. Make positive lab personnel and all your docs understand you use this drug.

THE ACTIVE INGREDIENTS IN ACXION PILLS

The essential active aspect in ACXION Pills is Phentermine hydrochloride. This compound acts as a stimulant at the vital fearful device, suppressing urge for food and increasing metabolism. ACXION Pills may additionally comprise different inactive elements that assist with the absorption and transport of the medication. Phentermine hydrochloride, as a sympathomimetic amine, works by mimicking the consequences of neurotransmitters in the mind. It stimulates the release of norepinephrine, a hormone that controls starvation alerts. By increasing the levels of norepinephrine, ACXION Pills successfully lessen your appetite and make you sense happy with smaller portions of food. Furthermore, ACXION Pills additionally increase your metabolism, main to expanded calorie burning. This metabolic enhancement helps you burn greater fats and attain weight reduction greater efficaciously. By combining urge for food suppression with an expanded metabolism, ACXION Pills offer a comprehensive method to weight management. It is crucial to observe that ACXION Pills have to only be used below the steering of a healthcare professional. They are commonly prescribed for people with a frame mass index (BMI) of 30 or better, or for those with a BMI of 27 or better who have additional danger factors along with high blood strain or diabetes. Before starting any weight reduction medicinal drug, it's far important to discuss with your medical doctor to decide if ACXION Pills are the proper preference for you. They will assess your overall fitness, examine potential dangers and blessings, and offer customized steering that will help you achieve your weight reduction goals thoroughly and efficaciously. In conclusion, ACXION Pills, or Phentermine, are prescription urge for food suppressants which can aid in weight reduction by using lowering hunger and increasing metabolism. Their lively component, Phentermine hydrochloride, acts as a stimulant at the significant anxious system, curbing cravings and promoting satiety. However, it is essential to keep in mind that these pills must simplest be used under medical supervision. Always talk over with your healthcare expert to decide the high-quality approach to your weight reduction adventure.

THE BENEFITS OF ACXION PILLS

ACXION Pills provide numerous blessings for individuals suffering with weight loss. When blended with a wholesome weight loss program and normal exercising, ACXION Pills can be an effective tool for weight loss. Studies have shown that ACXION Pills can assist people lose a median of five% to 10% in their body weight within some months. This weight reduction can have full-size fitness benefits, which includes lowering the danger of obesity-associated situations like diabetes, excessive blood pressure, and heart disorder. ACXION Pills no longer only assist with weight reduction but also provide an electricity improve. Phentermine stimulates the release of positive neurotransmitters within the brain, resulting in multiplied electricity stages. This can be mainly beneficial for folks who conflict with fatigue or lack of motivation at some point of their weight reduction journey.

Weight Loss and ACXION

Weight loss is a not unusual goal for plenty individuals, and ACXION Pills can play a huge role in attaining that purpose. By combining ACXION Pills with a healthful weight loss plan and normal exercising, people can enjoy considerable weight loss consequences. The lively component in ACXION Pills, phentermine, works by suppressing urge for food and increasing metabolism, making it less difficult for people to paste to their food regimen and burn energy.

Studies have proven that ACXION Pills can assist people lose an average of five% to ten% of their body weight inside some months. This weight reduction is not most effective aesthetically eye-catching however also has severa health benefits. Excess weight can put stress on the frame, main to numerous obesity-related situations which include diabetes, high blood strain, and heart disorder. By shedding those extra pounds, individuals can notably reduce their risk of growing these conditions and improve their universal fitness.

Furthermore, the weight reduction performed thru ACXION Pills can boost individuals' self-esteem and self assurance. Losing weight can enhance frame picture and growth emotions of self confidence, main to a extra advantageous outlook on life. This newfound self belief will have a ripple impact, positively impacting different regions of lifestyles, inclusive of relationships, profession, and average happiness.

Energy Boosting Properties of ACXION

One of the introduced blessings of ACXION Pills is the power improve they offer. Phentermine, the lively factor in ACXION Pills, stimulates the discharge of positive neurotransmitters within the mind, resulting in expanded electricity ranges. This can be particularly beneficial for those who conflict with fatigue or lack of motivation in the course of their weight reduction journey.

With accelerated energy ranges, individuals can tackle their daily duties with extra vigour and exuberance. They may additionally find it simpler to engage in physical sports and workout, which might be crucial for weight reduction. Regular exercise now not best enables burn energy but also improves cardiovascular fitness, strengthens muscle mass, and complements standard nicely-being.

In addition to bodily power, ACXION Pills also can provide mental clarity and cognizance. The accelerated neurotransmitter activity inside the brain can decorate cognitive characteristic, making it easier for people to live focused on their weight loss goals and make healthier picks. This mental readability can extend past weight loss and definitely effect different regions of life, which includes work, relationships, and private boom. It's crucial to notice that whilst ACXION Pills can provide an power raise, it is critical to preserve a balanced lifestyle. Adequate relaxation, hydration, and vitamins are crucial for universal well-being and ought to be prioritized alongside using ACXION Pills.

THE END